Dermatitis Herpetiformis: A Concise Guide to Causes, Tests and Treatment Options

JF Smithson, MA

John P. Barrons, MD (Ed.)

Contents

Introduction

Dermatitis herpetiformis (DH) is a rare skin disorder that is chronic; symptoms can come and go for years unless treated. It was first described in medical journals in 1884 by Louis Duhring, an American dermatologist. It wasn't until 1967 that a connection was made between DH and celiac disease intolerance to gluten). However, the exact causal mechanism is not known even today.

DH is also known as Brocq-Duhring Disease, Dermatitis Multiformis, and Duhring Disease. Dermatitis herpetiformis gets its name because the skin lesions have a similar appearance to herpes. However, there is no relation between DH and the herpes virus itself.

The disease tends to affect men slightly more than women; for every 3 men that get DH, 2 women are affected. The condition is rare and thought to occur in about 1 in 2500 people. It is usually seen in adults over 20 years of age, with most cases being middle-aged adults. It is rarely seen in children although some cases have been reported in the medical literature. Caucasians are more likely to suffer from DH; it is rarer in Asian populations.

The exact cause of DH isn't known but the vast majority of patients (around three quarters) also have celiac disease. This involves the inability to digest gluten (a protein found in wheat and related grains like barley and rye). Current thinking is that DH is a manifestation on the skin of celiac disease. However you don't always have to have digestive issues to get DH; around 15 to 25 percent of people diagnosed with the condition do not have any digestive symptoms.

What is Celiac Disease?

Celiac disease is an autoimmune disorder that damages the small intestine and interferes with the body's absorption of nutrients. A person with celiac should not consume any product with gluten. This includes foods with wheat, rye or barely and many other products like medicines, vitamins and lip products. If gluten is consumed, the body responds by damaging parts of the small intestine called the villi, which is the part of the intestine that absorbs nutrients. Thus, people with celiac disease may suffer from vitamin deficiencies.

Dermatitis herpetiformis is characterized by groups of itchy blisters on the skin called *pruritic blisters* ("pruritic" means itching) and raised lesions on the skin, called papules. It can also cause red bumps, similar to hives. Blisters tend to be very small, with the largest blisters reaching about 1 cm in size. In the first stage of the disease, you may notice a slight skin discoloration. The next stage is characterized by the formation of bumps and blisters. In the last stage, the lesions heal. However, skin discoloration commonly remains; these areas may be lighter or darker than your normal skin tone.

The most common areas where pruritic blisters and raised lesions appear are on the buttocks, elbows, knees and shoulder blades. However, lesions and blisters may also appear on the neck and head. Half of people with DH also have discolored, darkened skin pigmentation around the areas where the blisters and lesions are.

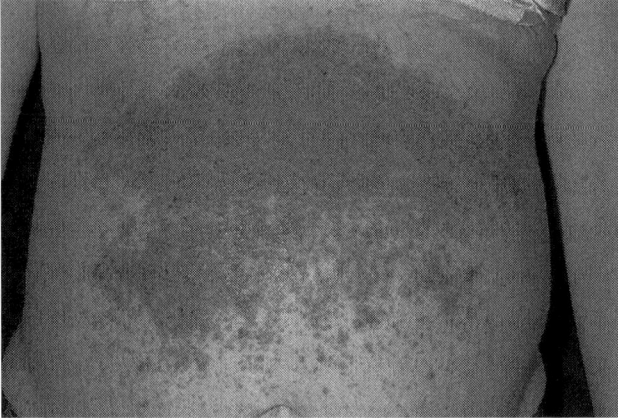

The characteristic skin rash of dermatitis herpetiformis. Image: Dermnet.com

Symptoms of the disease appear gradually, usually during adulthood. The skin becomes intensely red with red lesions, fluid filled lesions and raised lesions (bumps) on the skin on both sides of the body. The lesions can be extremely itchy, like bug bites. Often, you might find you *have* to scratch – the itching is so intense it might be hard for you to think about anything else but the relief that comes from scratching. The intense stinging, burning and itching may keep patients awake at night.

DH can look like eczema, leading to the condition often being misdiagnosed by general practitioners. However, the treatment for DH is vastly different from the treatment for eczema. Additionally, people with DH often have celiac and other autoimmune disorders like thyroid disease.

What is Thyroid Disease?

Many patients with DH also have thyroid disease. People with celiac disease are four times more likely to develop autoimmune thyroiditis. Autoimmune thyroiditis (Hashimoto's thyroiditis) is the most common type of thyroid disease. When the thyroid gland enlarges, it doesn't produce enough hormones. The body uses energy slower than it should, which often means weight gain and difficulty in losing weight. Graves disease is the most common cause of hyperthyroidism. It is rare in comparison to autoimmune thyroiditis. The thyroid produces too many hormones and then the body uses energy faster than it should, leading to unexpected weight loss along with other symptoms.

A gluten-free diet may help treat hypothyroidism. In particular, you may be able to decrease the amount of medication you take after your small intestine heals and your body's ability to absorb nutrients improves.

Although the development of DH can be alarming, the skin disorder can be treated simply. A gluten-free diet is usually recommended, along with an antibiotic called dapsone. Without treatment, there is a significant risk of developing intestinal cancer. DH is usually a lifelong condition. Rarely, remission can occur – typically in 10 to 20 percent of patients.

Diagnosis

The first step in a diagnosis is to visit a dermatologist. DH is commonly misdiagnosed by general practitioners, so it's important to visit a specialist if you suspect you have DH.

Your dermatologist will conduct a physical examination. If the dermatologist notices unusual skin features, this often suggests a different diagnosis. For example, plaques -- broad, large papules – on the skin may indicate psoriasis (a condition where skin cells grow too quickly), burrows between the fingers may be a result of scabies (an itchy skin rash caused by a mite) or blistering in the mouth may suggest pemphigus (another rare skin disorder that causes blisters).

Immunoglobulin A

Antibodies protect the body from foreign invaders (antigens) like bacteria and viruses in these areas by binding to the antigen. The antibody can neutralize the target directly or signal other parts of the immune system to attack the invader.

In DH, an antibody called Immunoglobulin A (IgA) is deposited in the skin. This antibody is normally found in breathing passages, the digestive tract, vagina, ears and eyes, saliva, tears and blood.

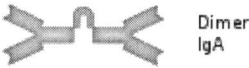

Dimer
IgA

IgA is not normally found in the skin, so a positive finding for IgA can help to confirm dermatitis herpetiformis. This can be detected with a skin biopsy. However, other conditions can cause IgA deposits in the skin so a positive skin biopsy isn't the only tool your dermatologist will use to make a diagnosis.

The type of biopsy used to detect IgA is called a punch biopsy.

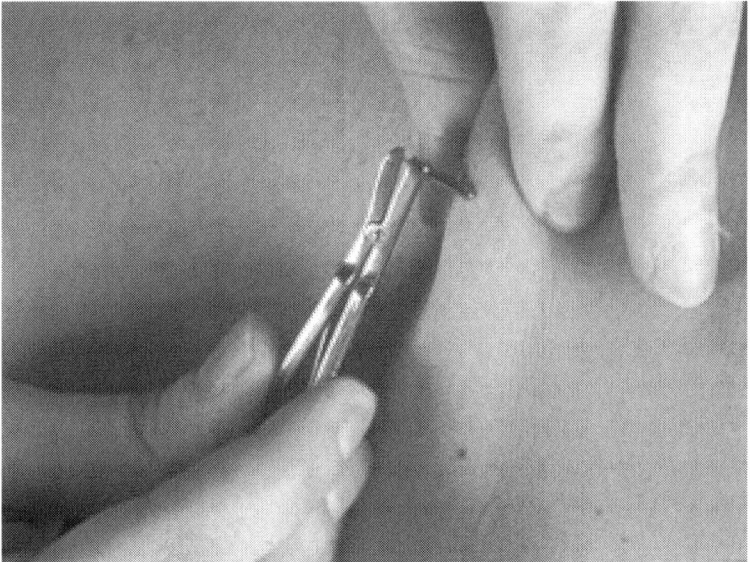

Punch biopsy. Image: CDC.gov.

A skin biopsy takes about 15 minutes, including cleaning around the area to be biopsied and closing (suturing) the wound. You will receive some type of numbing medicine (anesthetic) before your skin biopsy. The anesthetic will be given with a thin needle. The medication should numb the area so that you do not feel pain during the biopsy. Your doctor will remove a small round piece of skin (usually the size of a pencil eraser) using a sharp, hollow instrument with a circular blade. The blades are small—between 2mm and 8mm in diameter. If a large sample is taken, the area may be closed with stitches. A dressing or adhesive bandage will be placed on the area. The biopsy is sent to the lab and technicians will look for the presence of IgA. The biopsy should be performed in an area of unaffected skin near a lesion, because the actual lesions often do not have traces of IgA.

Healing of the wound takes a few weeks to two months. The biopsy will cause a small scar, which may be raised. You'll be given instructions for wound care before you leave the physician's office, but in general you should not touch the biopsy site unless your hands are clean. You can wash the site with soap and water (or shampoo, if the site is on your scalp). Make sure you rinse the site well, pat dry and cover the site with a clean dressing or bandage. The scar will fade gradually. After about two years, the scar is permanent and may be a pink, white, or brown color.

A lab technician will examine the skin under the microscope. If the biopsy has been taken from a section of normal skin adjacent to the affected area, a technique called direct immunofluorescence (light microscopy with a fluorescence microscope) will show granular IgA deposits in the upper dermis. The dermis is the inner layer of the skin.

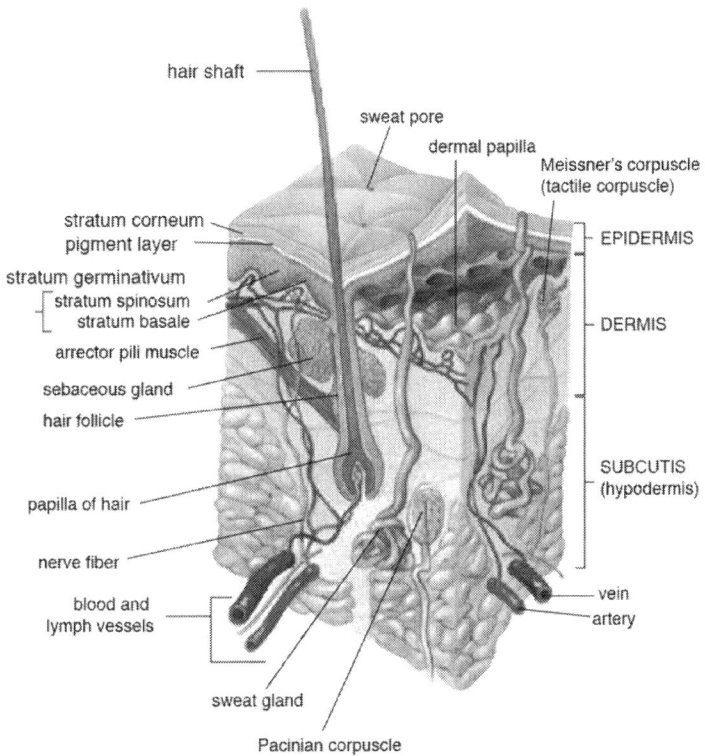

hair shaft

sweat pore

dermal papilla

Meissner's corpuscle
(tactile corpuscle)

stratum corneum
pigment layer

EPIDERMIS

stratum germinativum
stratum spinosum
stratum basale

DERMIS

arrector pili muscle

sebaceous gland

hair follicle

SUBCUTIS
(hypodermis)

papilla of hair

nerve fiber

blood and
lymph vessels

vein

artery

sweat gland

Pacinian corpuscle

Layers of the skin.

If the biopsy site is the affected skin (not recommended for diagnosis), the technician may notice small abscesses (called microabscesses) which contain white blood cells (neutrophils or eosinophils). However, the intense itching a patient has may mean the skin has been stripped and there may be no white blood cells in the area.

Blood tests

Blood tests for other antibodies--antiendomysial and anti-tissue transglutaminase antibodies—aid the diagnostic process. These antibodies are often found in people with dermatitis herpetiformis and celiac disease. Recent research has shown that many DH patients have an unusual presence of epidermal transglutaminase in their skin ("epidermal" means the outermost layers of the skin). Although it isn't understood exactly why patients have this enzyme presence in their skin, it's hoped that this finding will lead to figuring out the cause of DH.

Tests for Celiac Disease

If you have a positive test for DH, it's very likely your doctor will want to test you for celiac because of the high probability you also have celiac disease. Any tests need to be performed while you are still eating gluten. A physical examination and a blood test for antibodies can indicate celiac disease. However, a diagnosis is confirmed with a biopsy of your small intestine.

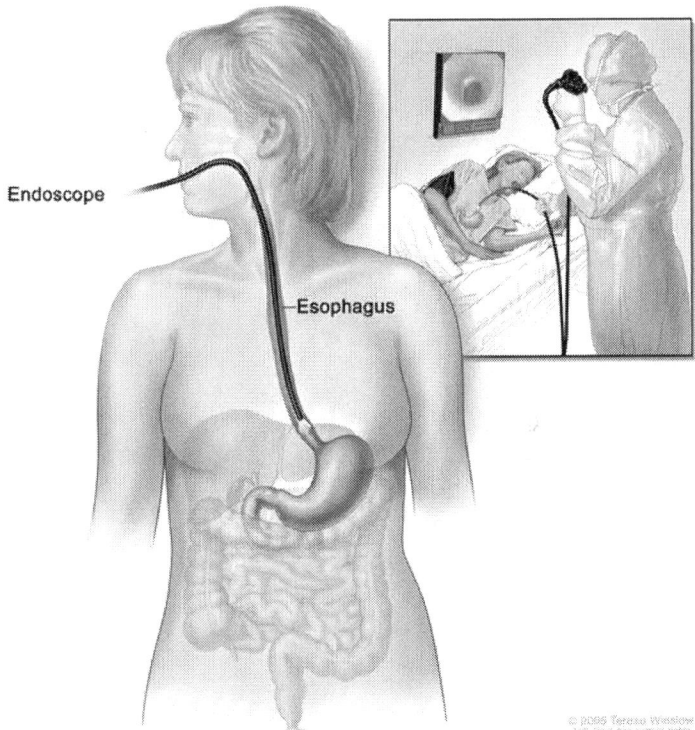

Esophagoscopy

Endoscope

Esophagus

The biopsy for celiac disease takes about 10-15 minutes. During a biopsy, a physician will use a thin long tube with a camera (called an endoscope) to take a small piece of tissue from your intestine. This tissue is then examined in the lab. Adults are normally prescribed a sedative for the procedure; children are usually given general anesthesia.

The physician will insert the endoscope into your mouth and down the esophagus (the passageway to your stomach). Once in the stomach, the physician will use the camera to find the opening to your small intestine (the duodenum). Once in the small intestine, the physician will insert a tiny surgical instrument into the endoscopy tube, which they will use to take a small piece of tissue from your small intestine. After the biopsy, a pathologist will examine the tissue for celiac disease.

Causes

DH develops when there is an environmental trigger. Essentially, the disease usually develops as a result of eating gluten – a protein found in cereals like wheat, rye, and barley. In a few rare cases, the condition has been implicated as being induced by drugs, including ibuprofen, fluriprofen (Tousignant) and leuprolide acetate.

The dermatitis herpetiformis rash is caused when gluten combines with the IgA antibody. Together the gluten and IgA enter the blood stream and circulate around the body, eventually ending up in the small blood vessels in the skin, where they create a clog. The clog attracts white blood cells (neutrophils), which release chemicals called complements. The complements cause the dermatitis herpetiformis rash. According to the American Osteopathic College of Dermatology, iodine is required for this reaction to occur, so if you have DH you should avoid using Iodized salt.

Many studies in recent years have tried to find out exactly why eating gluten causes the development of DH lesions. Although scientists think there is a link, they have to date been unable to determine exactly how that link operates (Sardy).

Genetics

What is known for sure is that DH has a genetic component. According to the British Association of Dermatologists, 1 in 10 people with DH has a family history of either DH or of celiac disease. That means DH runs in some families, although just because you don't have DH or celiac in your family does not mean that you don't have either disease.

The genetic component through to be involved with DH and celiac is called Human Leukocyte Antigen (HLA). The HLA complex helps your body to tell the difference between your own proteins and those proteins produced by a foreign invader, like viruses or bacteria. When there is a defect in the HLA complex (what geneticists call a *mutation),* your body may think that your own proteins are foreign invaders.

Essentially, your body attacks itself, causing immune system problems like DH or Celiac disease.

Two specific genes are thought to be involved with the development of DH: HLA DQ2 and HLA DQ8. In one study (Spurkland), 86% of people with DH carried the HLA DQ2 allele (variation) and 12% carried the HLA DQ8 allele. Many studies in the 70s and 80s suggested other gene involvement for DH and Celiac, including: HLA-A1, HLA-B8, and HLA-DR3. However, later research could not confirm any of those findings.

How do Gene Mutations Happen?

Gene mutations that are passed from one of your parents are called hereditary mutations or germline mutations. The word "germline" is used because egg and sperm cells are also called germ cells. It's also possible for a mutation to occur in either an egg or a sperm. In other words, a parent doesn't have the mutations but one of their germ cells does. These mutations are known as "de novo" mutations; de novo means "new". A third type of mutation is called an acquired or somatic mutation. These types of mutations can occur if a mistake is made when the DNA copies itself during development. Acquired mutations are not passed on to the next generation. DH can be de novo, germline, or acquired mutations.

Our bodies contain about 20,000 genes, which are carried on 46 structures called chromosomes. These chromosomes come as 22 pairs of XX (one from each parent), and two sex chromosomes, XX for a girl and XY for a boy... Each chromosome has a small arm (P for the French "Petit) and a long Q arm. HLA can be found on a specific area of chromosome 6.

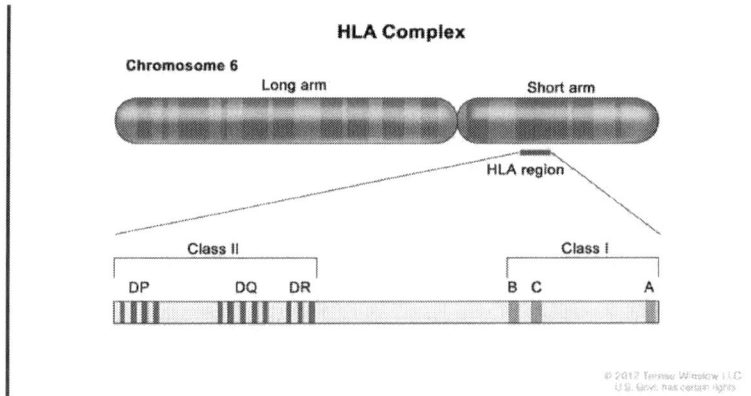

HLA Complex

Chromosome 6

Long arm — Short arm

HLA region

Class II — Class I

DP — DQ DR — B C — A

© 2012 Terese Winslow LLC
U.S. Govt. has certain rights

Human chromosome 6 showing the long and short arms of chromosome 6. The HLA region is shown on the short arm.

At the time of writing, there isn't a genetic test available for finding out if you have an HLA mutation for DH or celiac. It is technically possible to perform the test, but it would be very cost prohibitive (running into the thousands of dollars) and it would not aid in the diagnostic process: the skin biopsy for DH is more effective and cheaper for diagnostic purposes.

Related disorders

Many disorders cause symptoms that are similar to dermatitis herpetiformis. The National Institutes of health estimates that "over 95%" of DH cases are misdiagnosed, mostly because of non-dermatologists attempting to diagnose the disease. It isn't known exactly to what extent the disease is misdiagnosed, although celiac disease has long been recognized to be an often misdiagnosed disorder as well.

Linear IgA Disease

Linear IgA disease is a rare disease that causes blisters on the skin of adults. Like DH, IgA is also deposited in the skin. However, unlike DH, there is no link to celiac disease and the condition is not hereditary. It isn't known what causes linear IgA disease.

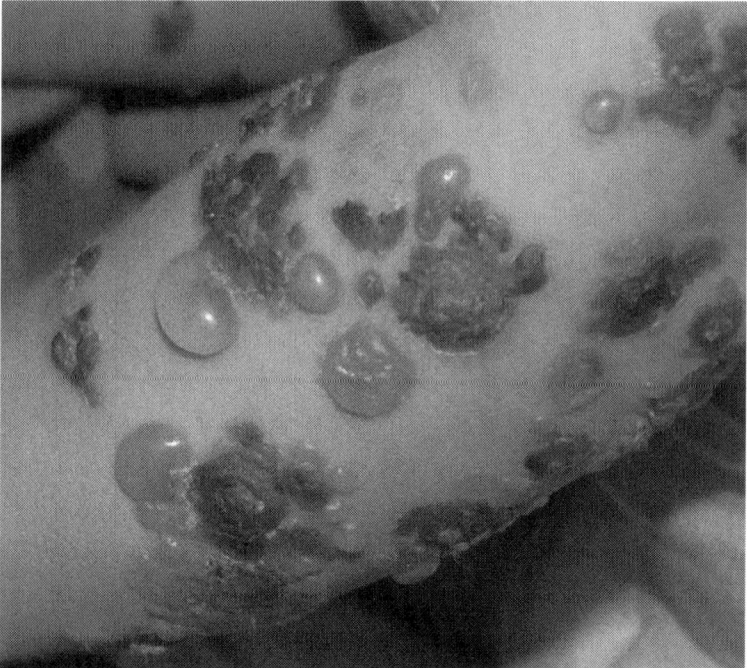

Bullous pemphigoid

Bullous pemphigoid causes redness, irritation and redness on the skin. In severe cases, there are multiple blisters (bullae). These blisters are usually found on the arms legs and middle of the body. Around a third of patients also have blisters in the mouth. Treatment is usually the use of corticosteroids although in some cases chemotherapy may be necessary to suppress the immune system. The condition normally resolves in a few years. The cause of the condition is not known.

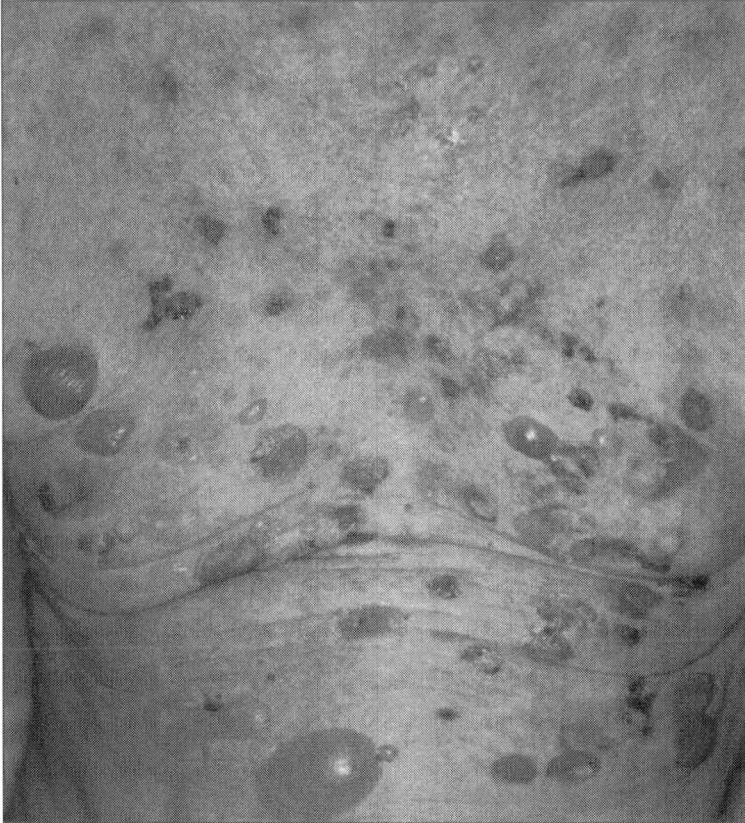

Pemphigus

Pemphigus is a rare autoimmune disorder that causes blisters, which can cover a very large area of skin. The condition is diagnosed with a skin biopsy and the finding that the upper part of the epidermis is sloughing off, leaving a bottom layer of cells on the floor of the blister that have a tombstone-like appearance. In addition, antibodies are found. However, while IgA deposits are found in DH, a different antibody called IgG is found instead. Pemphigus can be fatal if left untreated, due to massive infection from the sores.

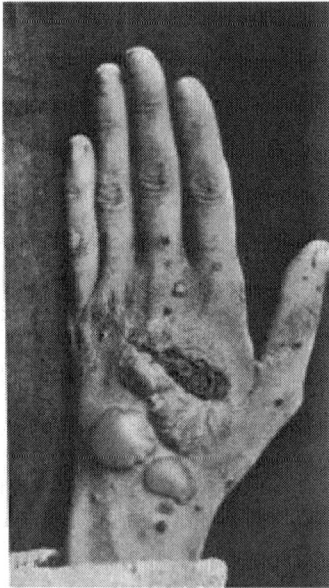

Erythema multiforme

Erythema multiforme causes red, itchy pink-red blotches on the skin. A skin biopsy in most cases will show deposits of an antibody called IgM in the skin. Most cases resolve in around 7-10 days. In severe cases, it can be a life-threatening disease.

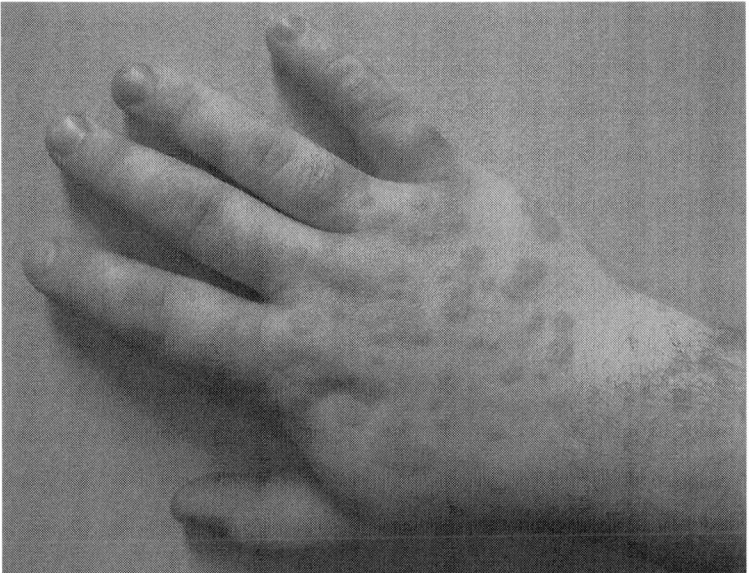

Epidermolytic hyperkeratosis

Epidermolytic hyperkeratosis involves the clumping of keratin filaments. Keratin is a structural material that makes up the outer layer of skin. The disorder is present at birth, causing babies to have red skin and blisters.

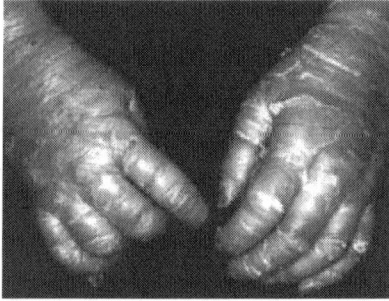

Epidermolysis bullosa

Epidermolysis bullosa is an inherited skin disorder that results in a defect in anchoring the outer layer of skin (the epidermis) to the inner layer (the dermis). The result is very fragile skin. In severe cases, it can be lethal.

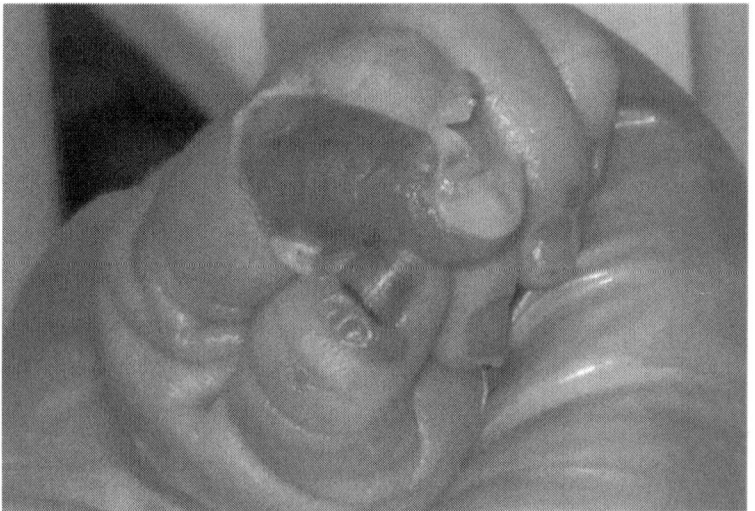

Treatment

Both the DH rash and the enteropathy (inflammation in the intestine) improve after a gluten-free diet (Bolotin). However, a gluten-free diet can take many months to resolve symptoms. Therefore, if you have DH your physician will probably recommend a drug called dapsone. If you take dapsone, you should see an improvement in your rash in as little as 1-2 days.

Dapsone comes in tablet form and is usually taken once a day or three times a week. According to the National Institutes of Health you should take the following precautions before taking dapsone:

- Tell your doctor and pharmacist if you have any drug allergies, especially dapsone, naphthalene, niridazole, nitrofurantoin, phenylhydrazine, primaquine and sulfa drugs.
- Tell your doctor and pharmacist about every medication you are taking (including over the counter drugs), especially aminobenzoate potassium (Potaba), aminobenzoic acid, clofazimine (Lamprene), didanosine (Videx), probenecid (Benemid), pyrimethamine (Daraprim), rifampin (Rifadin), trimethoprim (Bactrim, Cotrim, Septra), or vitamins. Note that nonsteroidal anti-inflammatory drugs (NSAIDs) like aspirin, ibuprofen and naproxen can make DH worse and are not recommended if you have the condition.
- Tell your doctor if you have or have ever had anemia or liver disease.
- Tell your doctor if you are pregnant, plan to become pregnant, or are breast-feeding. If you become pregnant while taking dapsone, call your doctor.
- Plan to avoid unnecessary or prolonged exposure to sunlight and to wear protective clothing, sunglasses, and sunscreen.

Dapsone may make your skin sensitive to sunlight.

Most side effects are mild, including vomiting, headache, nausea, loss of appetite, nervousness and trouble sleeping. Dapsone can cause serious side effects, including the destruction of red blood cells (hemolysis). About 20 percent of patients taking dapsone will get hemolysis. Although rare, aplastic anemia can also occur and can be fatal. Therefore, if you're taking dapsone it's recommended you have periodic blood tests to monitor for any changes in your blood counts.

You should call your doctor immediately if you experience any of the following symptoms while taking dapsone:

- Back, leg or stomach pain
- Bluish fingernails, lips or skin
- Difficulty breathing
- Fever
- Itching, dryness, scaling or peeling of skin that is unusual for you
- Loss of appetite
- Loss of hair
- Mood or mental changes including depression and mania.
- Numbness, tingling, pain, burning or weakness in your hands or feet

- Pale skin
- Rash
- Skin rash that is unusual for you
- Sore throat
- Unusual bleeding or bruising
- Unusual tiredness or weakness
- Yellowing of the skin or eyes

Some people with dermatitis herpetiformis who also have celiac disease may be able to discontinue dapsone use by following a strict gluten-free diet for at least 6 to 12 months.

The Gluten-Free Diet

A gluten-free diet means that you do not eat foods with wheat, rye and barley. The most common products which contain these grains are pasta, bread and cereal. Almost all commercial breakfast cereals contain gluten although there are a couple of gluten-free ones on the market (including gluten-free Rice Krispies). Look for products on the shelves labeled gluten-free. Many gluten-free products are widely available including bread, pancake mixes, cereals and processed foods. Organic and natural food stores are more likely to carry gluten-free foods, although many mainstream stores are carrying more and more of these products as celiac disease becomes more recognized. The popularity of the gluten-free diet for people who want to lose weight (although it's debated on if this actually works or not) has also resulted in an abundance of gluten-free products.

That said, just because it's labeled as gluten-free doesn't mean it's good for you. To make up for the loss of texture and taste that gluten provides foods, many products contain excess fats, sugars and other unwanted ingredients. You may be better off sticking to a relatively simple diet – think about shopping around the edges of the grocery store: meat, fish, fruits, vegetables and dairy. In general, you should avoid eating at restaurants as trace amounts of gluten are found in almost all restaurant foods.

The following list of foods should be a starting point for your diet. Make sure to check all labels: food manufacturers are required to list wheat as a possible allergen on food labels. However, they are *not* required to label other sources of gluten (such as barley and rye). Therefore you should read *all* food labels carefully. If you aren't sure what an ingredient is, avoid eating the product until you find out what the source of that product is.

Allowed Foods:

- Amaranth
- Arrowroot
- Buckwheat
- Cassava
- Corn
- Dairy (check labels)

- Fish
- Flax
- Fruit
- Indian Rice Grass
- Job's Tears
- Legumes (Beans)
- Meat
- Millet
- Nuts
- Quinoa
- Rice
- Sago
- Seeds
- Sorghum
- Soy
- Tapioca
- Teff
- Vegetables
- Wild Rice
- Yucca

Food to Avoid

- Wheat: including einkorn, emmer, spelt, kamut wheat starch, wheat bran, wheat germ, cracked wheat, hydrolyzed wheat protein
    - Barley
    - Rye
    - Triticale (a cross between wheat and rye)

- Bromated flour
- Durum flour
- Enriched flour
- Farina graham flour
- Phosphated flour
- Plain flour
- Self-rising flour
- Semolina
- White flour

Foods that may contain hidden gluten:

- Bouillon cubes
- Brown rice syrup
- Candy
- Chips/potato chips
- Cold cuts, hot dog, salami, sausage
- Communion wafers
- French fries
- Gravy
- Imitation fish and crab
- Matzo
- Rice mixes
- Sauces
- Seasoned tortilla chips
- Self-basting turkey
- Soups
- Soy sauce
- Vegetables in sauce

Source: National Institute of Diabetes and Digestive and Kidney Diseases (NIDDK), National Institutes of Health (NIH)

References

American Osteopathic College of Dermatology. Dermatitis Herpetiformis. http://www.aocd.org/?page=DermatitisHerpetifo

D. Bolotin and V. Petronic-Rosic, "Dermatitis herpetiformis: part II. Diagnosis, management, and prognosis," Journal of the American Academy of Dermatology, vol. 64, no. 6, pp. 1027–1033, 2011. View at Publisher · View at Google Scholar · View at Scopus

British Association of Dermatologists. Dermatitis Herpetiformis (Gluten Sensitivity). http://www.bad.org.uk/library-media%5Cdocuments%5CDermatitis%20Herpetiformis%20Update%20Jan%202013%20-%20lay%20reviewed%20Dec%202012.pdf

Grimwood, R. MD; Guevara, A. MD. Leuprolide Acetate–Induced Dermatitis Herpetiformis American Journal of Orthopedics. VOLUME 75, JANUARY 2005 49. National Institute of Diabetes and Digestive and Kidney Diseases (NIDDK), National Institutes of Health (NIH) Celiac Disease. http://digestive.niddk.nih.gov/DDISEASES/pubs/celiac/#table

Spurkland, G. Ingvarsson, E. S. Falk, I. Knutsen, L. M. Sollid, and E. Thorsby, "Dermatitis herpetiformis and celiac disease are both primarily associated with the HLA-DQ ($\alpha1*0501$, $\beta1*02$) or the HLA-DQ ($\alpha1*03$, $\beta1*0302$) heterodimers," Tissue Antigens, vol. 49, no. 1, pp. 29–34, 1997.

NIH Services USDoHaH. Celiac Disease Awareness Campaign of the National Institutes of Health. 2013.http://celiac.nih.gov/Dermatitis.aspx.

Tousignant J, Lafontaine N, Rochette L, et al. Dermatitis herpetiformis induced by nonsteroidal anti-inflammatory drugs. Int J Dermatol. 1993;33:199-200.

Images

IGA: Martin Brändli | Wikimedia Commons.

Linear IgA disease: Dermaamin.com.

Bullous pemphigoid: diseasespictures.com

Erythema Multiforme: James Heilman MD

Epidermolytic hyperkeratosis: Meduweb.com

Epidermolysis bullosa : JGSF.org

Made in the USA
San Bernardino, CA
19 March 2016

A PEOPLE AND A NATION

VOLUME I: TO 1877

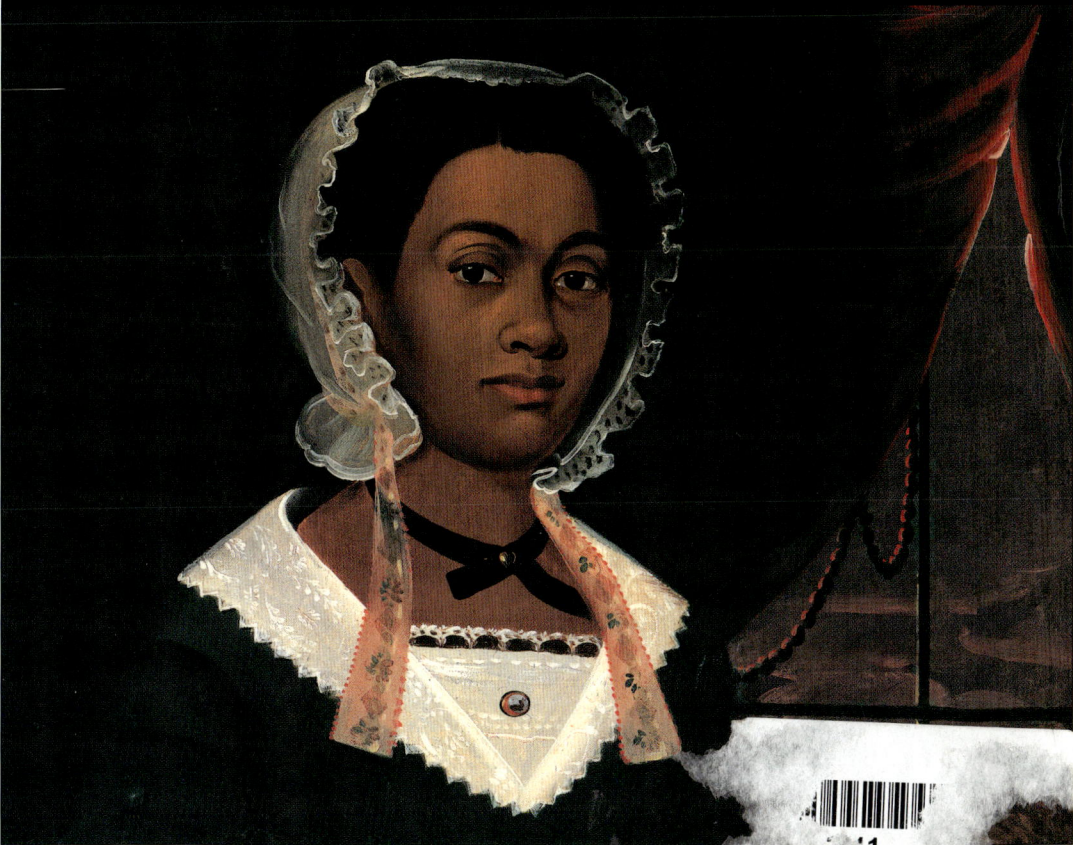

NORTON KATZMAN BLIGHT CHUDACOFF LOGEVALL BAILEY PATERSON TUTTLE